YOUR KNOWLEDGE HAS VALUE

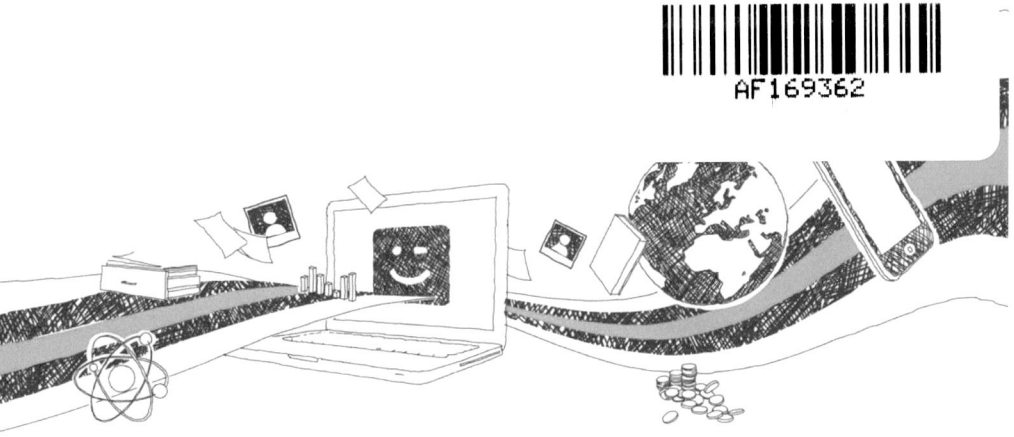

- We will publish your bachelor's and master's thesis, essays and papers

- Your own eBook and book - sold worldwide in all relevant shops

- Earn money with each sale

Upload your text at www.GRIN.com
and publish for free

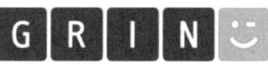

Bibliographic information published by the German National Library:

The German National Library lists this publication in the National Bibliography; detailed bibliographic data are available on the Internet at http://dnb.dnb.de .

This book is copyright material and must not be copied, reproduced, transferred, distributed, leased, licensed or publicly performed or used in any way except as specifically permitted in writing by the publishers, as allowed under the terms and conditions under which it was purchased or as strictly permitted by applicable copyright law. Any unauthorized distribution or use of this text may be a direct infringement of the author s and publisher s rights and those responsible may be liable in law accordingly.

Imprint:

Copyright © 2017 GRIN Verlag
Print and binding: Books on Demand GmbH, Norderstedt Germany
ISBN: 9783668622654

This book at GRIN:

https://www.grin.com/document/384368

Patrick Kimuyu

Review on Social Anxiety Disorder among Teenagers

GRIN Verlag

GRIN - Your knowledge has value

Since its foundation in 1998, GRIN has specialized in publishing academic texts by students, college teachers and other academics as e-book and printed book. The website www.grin.com is an ideal platform for presenting term papers, final papers, scientific essays, dissertations and specialist books.

Visit us on the internet:

http://www.grin.com/

http://www.facebook.com/grincom

http://www.twitter.com/grin_com

A Systematic Review on Social Anxiety Disorder in Teenagers

Name: Patrick Kimuyu

Contents

Abstract 3

Introduction 3

Etiology and Progression of Social Anxiety Disorder 5

Symptoms 6

Prevalence 7

Co-morbidity 9

Intervention 9

Treatment and Prognosis 10

How it Affects Patients, Families, and Society 11

Conclusion 11

References 13

Abstract

This research paper provides a literature review of social anxiety disorder among teenagers. In-depth research has been carried out on social anxiety disorder etiology and progression of the disorder, symptoms, prevalence, co-morbidity, a method of intervention (therapy), treatment and prognosis, and how it affects patients, families, and society. A critical analysis of the literature review shows that social anxiety disorder is an impairing disorder thus requiring both psysiological and medical treatment for effective results. The risk factors of the disorder are genetic factors, biological factors, neurological factors, and parental factors. Its symptoms include excessive fear, negative self evaluation, worry, and behavioral avoidance. Research has shown that this disorder is more prevalent in girls than boys. If diagnosed, social anxiety disorder can be treated by both physiological therapies and medical treatments which must be go together for effective results.

Introduction

Social anxiety disorder is one of the most debated anxiety disorders in psychology studies over the years because of its increasing prevalence among teenagers. Social anxiety disorder also known as social phobia is a persistent anxiety or fear of social situations way beyond the actual threat exposed by the situation (Turner, Beidel & Borden, 2001). These social situations are anxiety provoking thus resulting into fear among the individual. Some of the anxiety provoking situations include public speaking, being seen in public, eating while being observed, chatting with authoritative figures, starting conversations, talking in groups or teams, and meeting strangers (Fehm & Pelissolo, 2005).

Teenagers with social anxiety disorder tend to exhibit fear and anxiety when exposed to some of these social situations or performances. If these teenagers are at the center of attention, their anxiety is induced and in many cases, they tend to withdraw from these situations. The people with this disorder worry excessively before, during and after experiencing these situations because of the fear or worry that they might say or act something embarrassing or humiliating for instance, looking anxious, disrupting normal life, looking incompetent, shaking, sweating, and blushing(Beidel et al, 2007). As a result, the performance of the individual declines for instance, if in a work place, the individual functioning is impacted negatively. If at school, social anxiety disorder impairs their learning and at home, the quality of life and social relationship is impacted negatively because of the disruption of normal quality life (Baron & Kenny, 2006).

Majority of the teenagers with social anxiety disorder tend to misuse drugs and alcohol so as to alleviate depression and also reduce their anxiety. They also experience difficulties in getting employment and getting involved in marriages. In school, these teenagers have educational underachievement and this is according to a research in US which shows that 91 percent of teenagers with social anxiety disorder lack academic advancement because of the social phobic fears they have developed. That said; social anxiety disorder is an impairing disorder thus requiring a method of intervention (therapy), treatment and prognosis (Asher, Hymel & Renshaw, 2004).

Etiology and Progression of Social Anxiety Disorder

Etiology refers to the risk factors of the disorder. Social anxiety disorder has several risk factors which include genetic factors, neurobiological factors, biological factors, temperament, and parent factors. The most common risk factor is genetic factors. Research by kindler, Myers & Neale, (2001) on male twin pairs shows that there is a genetic component unique to social anxiety disorder with 13 percent of social fears being accounted for genetic components. This implies that teenagers with social anxiety disorder share a unique genetic encumbrance hence influencing for social fears. The same research has shown that there is a heritability estimate of 0.65 for social anxiety. Ollendick & Hirshfeld (2002) concur with the same findings by reporting estimates of 0.5 percent heritability estimate of social anxiety.

Neurological factors have also contributed to the prevalence of social anxiety disorder among teenagers. Research shows that when people are afraid, neurological techniques such as fMRI and PET result into increased amygdale (this is a set of neurons in the brain) which result into fear. Some people have more amygdale than others hence the differences in social fear. The other factor is temperament which is behavior inhibition found in teenagers and children with social anxiety disorder. Fearfulness, cautiousness, and avoidance behavior are typical behaviors witnessed in people with behavior inhibition. These people activate amygdale faster thus resulting into social fear (Kendler et al, 2001). As regards biological factors, research has shown that teenagers with social anxiety disorder have higher physiological arousal and anxiety sensitivity. Parental factors have also contributed to the high prevalence of social anxiety disorders. Research has shown that there is a reciprocal relationship between child and parent behavior as regards social anxiety (Tillfors et al, 2001). Anxious children have higher chances of having anxious parents and their behaviors are characterized with avoidance and anxiety. Due to the genetic makeup, a parent with a social anxiety disorder is more likely to have an offspring with social anxiety disorder. This is according to a research by Merikangas & Avenevoli (2000) who found that the risk for anxiety disorder in the offspring of a parent with the anxiety disorder is 3.5 times that of a non-anxious parent.

Symptoms

Social anxiety disorder is characterized with fear of social situations implying that teenagers when exposed to social situations such as public speaking develop physical symptoms such as trembling and blushing and this will have an impact on their performance. They also develop cognitive symptoms such as negative self evaluation, worry, and behavioral avoidance. For instance, in group meeting, teenagers with social anxiety disorder will less evaluate themselves and in many cases, they do not get actively involved in decision making and this will always have an impact on their performance. They develop fear to speak in groups and in meeting implying that their decisions might not be considered. They also develop behavioral avoidance whereby they do not mingle with others if in a workplace or at school (Adams et al, 2008).

Owing to their increased fear to form social relationships with others for instance, at school and at work, research has shown that these teenagers have loneliness and low social support. They have perceived burdensome and thwarted belongings and this might result into suicidal idealation (Hofmann & Asnaani, 2010). According to Joiners interpersonal theory of suicide, teenagers with social anxiety disorder have increased thoughts of suicidal attempts because of enhanced loneliness and low social support from friends and family members. They tend to be isolated from others because of their fear to mingle with others and this in many times results into suicidal behavior. Thwarted belongingness encompasses a feeling of loneliness and isolation among teenagers with the disorder (Groholt et al, 2000). They also develop a perception that they lack mutual supportive relationships and they also perceive that their lives have become a burdensome to themselves and the society too. The teenage stage or adolescence stage is marked with increased social relationship from family and friends and interpersonal difficulties such as loneliness and low social support from friends and families in many cases become problematic to teenagers with social anxiety disorder (Calsyn, Winter & Burger, 2005).

During the teenage stage, social anxiety disorder is impairing for instance, increased avoidance from friends, peers, and family members. 17 percent of the teenagers with social anxiety disorder avoid social situations for instance, group meetings and discussions and this result into academic underachievement. In a sample of 784 teenagers in the US with social anxiety disorder, two thirds of these teenagers (or 68 percent) were bullied in school because they cannot react back to social situations (Gunnell et al, 2008).

Prevalence

Social anxiety disorder has high prevalence among teenagers. In the United States for instance, the prevalence of the disorder among teenagers is higher approximately at 12 percent of the population compared with 6 percent of teenagers with generalized social disorders. Social anxiety disorder has high prevalence among teenagers compared with other social disorders such as obsessive compulsive disorder with a prevalence of 2 percent, post-traumatic stress disorder with a prevalence of 7 percent, and panic disorder with a prevalence of 5 percent in the United States. Research in the US also shows that social anxiety disorder is more prevalent among girls than boys (the disorder is twice as prevalence among girls as it is in boys). The estimated lifetime prevalence of the disorder in twelve month prevalence is 7.1 percent (Gunnell et al, 2008). A further research by Fehm and Pelissolo (2005) in a critical overview of 23 prevalence studies shows that in Europe 6.6 percent of the teenage population have social anxiety disorder. The twelve month prevalence of the disorder in Europe is 3 percent.

According to the National Co-morbidity Survey Replication-Adolescent Supplement in 2008 in the US, 0,123 teenagers aged between 13 to 18 years were surveyed for social anxiety disorder and the findings were that 8.6 percent of the teenagers surveyed had the social anxiety disorder, 55.8 percent had generalized social disorder while 44.2 percent had non-generalized social disorder. The same research also shows that high prevalence of social anxiety disorder is in the US compared to other countries such as Europe. According to Hofman, Asnaani & Hinton (2010), social anxiety disorder has cultural aspects with the high prevalence noticed in US and some Asian countries. The contributive factors towards this prevalence in US and Asian countries include gender role identification, gender roles, how self as an image is construed, individual perception of social norms, and collectivistic and individual orientation in society. Regarding gender roles and identification, the prevalence of social anxiety disorder is high among girls than boys. This is supported by research by Essau and Conradt (2000) who carried out a sample of 1035 teenagers and found that 2.1 percent of the female population sample had social anxiety disorder while 1.0 percent of the male population sample had the disorder. Regarding age of onset of social anxiety disorder, the disorder presents itself during late childhood and early adolescence. A study by Essau and Conradt (2000) on the prevalence of social anxiety disorder among three age groups shows that for ages between 12 and 13, the prevalence of the disorder was 0.5 percent; the ages between 14 to 15 had a prevalence of 2 percent while the ages between 16 to 17 had a prevalence of 2 percent. The findings, therefore, show that high social fear at 55.4 percent is found in the age group between 14 to 15 years while a higher social anxiety disorder was found in the age group between 15 to 17 years (Ranta & Marttunen, 2009).

Co-morbidity

According to the study by Turner, Beidel & Bordon, (2001) on 71 teenagers with social anxiety disorder, the generalized anxiety disorder is the most common co-morbidity disorder with a prevalence of 33 percent while simple phobia was found in 11 percent of the population sampled. Patients suffering from social anxiety disorder and another anxiety diagnosis are linked with high levels of depression and greater anxiety compared to patients only suffering from social anxiety disorder alone. This argument is in line with a research by Ranta & Martunem, (2009) who carried out a research on 350 teenagers with social anxiety disorder and the findings were that in 41 cases co-morbidity was witnessed with mood disorders such as high levels of depression. The research, therefore, concluded that one third of the teenagers with social anxiety disorder had another anxiety disorder during their lifetime. Examples of the most commonly observed anxiety disorders among the teenagers with social anxiety disorder were drug use disorder at 21 percent and 17.8 percent of oppositional defiant disorder. The same research also shows that co-morbidity rates are more with teenagers suffering from generalized subtype of social anxiety disorder. That said, co-morbidity is as a result of etiological relationships or diagnostic criteria artifacts (Burstein et al, 2011).

Intervention

The cognitive behavioral therapy is one of the most successful methods of intervention of social anxiety disorder. The cognitive behavioral therapy is composed of exposure therapy, social skills therapy, and cognitive restructuring therapy. The exposure therapy stands out as the best cognitive behavioral therapy whereby children and teenagers are exposed into various social and performance situations so as to reduce social anxiety (Davey, 2006). Cognitive restructuring, on the other hand, involves restructuring of negative thinking so as to suit the child maturity level. This ensures that the child focuses more on the positive components hence adjusting their mind to suit their vocabulary level (Edelmann & Baker, 2002). Enhanced social skills are also important for children and teenagers because social skills enhance their social relationships with others in school and at work. Their tutors need to focus more on the social skills so as to reduce the social phobic symptoms such as avoidance, fear, and arousal. If the tutors allow the social phobic symptoms to enhance such as fear and avoidance, they hinder the child from new learning and this result into poor performance in school and at work (Boergers & Spirito, 2003).

Other randomized controlled methods have being used to reduce social anxiety disorder among children and teenagers. For instance, social effectiveness training to reduce fears of interpersonal interactions and public performance fears. The social skills training, vivo exposure, and social effectiveness training helps teenagers with the disorder practice things such as telephone skills, how to join and participate in a group, how to listen and remember what others say, initiating and maintaining a conversation, and introducing oneself (Babiss & Gangwisch, 2009).

Treatment and Prognosis

A variety of treatments have been used to diagnose and treat social anxiety disorder among children and teenagers. A mental health professional provides a diagnosis for the disorder and an individual treatment plan begins. Other than the cognitive behavioral therapy, medications including selective serotonin reuptake inhibitors (SSRIs) have been used and they provide effective outcomes for instance, how people perceive events and situations in their daily lives thus developing skills to manage anxiety in the future. These medications are also known as antidepressants and they need to be taken under supervision of a medical doctor

(Ginsburg & Schlossberg, 2002). Medication is only recommended in situations when the child or teenager anxiety makes them unable to speak in certain situations for instance, in public. However, for the best results, these medications need to be taken alongside the psychological therapies such as the cognitive-behavioral therapy. A point to note is that there is no single medication for social anxiety disorder because what works for a certain person might not work for the other person implying that any form of medication whether physiological or medical should be tailored towards the individual needs of the patient. It is always important to ask the medical doctors to explain why a particular treatment is recommended and the other available options for the best treatment (Gallagher, Rabian & McCloskey, 2004).

How it Affects Patients, Families, and Society

Social anxiety disorder has huge effects to patients, families, and the society. For instance, as regards patient's effects, the patient has increased risk for drug and alcohol abuse, depression, and suicidal attempts. It disrupts family life because of lack of mutual relationship and communication, limit work efficiency and also reduce self-esteem (Epkins, 2002). People with the disorder in many cases have few or no social relationships hence disrupting families. It is also economically devastating to the society because these patients underperform both in school and at work. They experience difficulties getting a job and also finishing school thus affecting their living standards in the future (Alfano et al, 2009).

Conclusion

In conclusion, social anxiety disorder is an impairing disorder with huge impacts on the patient, family, and the society at large. It is a disabling disorder which is characterized by excessive self consciousness and overwhelming anxiety in social situations for instance, public speaking. Some of its symptoms include excessive fear, negative self evaluation, worry, and behavioral avoidance. Research has shown that this disorder is more prevalent in girls than boys and some of its risk factors include genetic factors, biological factors, parental factors, and neurological factors. If diagnosed, social anxiety disorder can be treated by both physiological therapies and medical treatments which must be go together for effective results.

References

Adams, G. R., Openshaw, D. K., Bennion, L., Mills, T., & Noble, S. (2008). Loneliness in late adolescence: a social skills training study. *Journal of Adolescent Research, 3,* 81–96.

Alfano, C. A., Pina, A. A., Villalta, I. K., Beidel, D. C., Ammerman, R. T., & Crosby, L. E. (2009). Mediators and moderators of outcome in the behavioral treatment of childhood social phobia. *Journal of the American Academy of Child and Adolescent Psychiatry, 48,* 945–953.

Asher, S. R., Hymel, S., & Renshaw, P. D. (2004). Loneliness in children. *Child Development, 55,* 1456–1464.

Babiss, L. A., & Gangwisch, J. E. (2009). Sports participation as a protective factor against depression and suicidal ideation in adolescents as mediated by self-esteem and social support. *Journal of Developmental and Behavioral Pediatrics, 30,* 376–384.

Baron, R. M., & Kenny, D. A. (2006). The moderator-mediator variable distinction in social psychological research: conceptual, strategic, and statistical considerations. *Journal of Personality and Social Psychology, 6,* 1173–1182.

Beidel, D. B., Turner, S. M., Young, B. J., Ammerman, R. T., Sallee, F. R., & Crosby, L. (2007). Psychopathology of adolescent social phobia. *Journal of Psychopathology and Behavioral Assessment, 29,* 47–54.

Boergers, J., & Spirito, A. (2003). *Follow-up studies of child and adolescent suicide attempters. In R. A. King & A. Apter (Eds.), Suicide in children and adolescents.* New York: Cambridge University Press.

Burstein, M., He, J.-P., Kattan, G., Albano, A. M., Avenevoli, S., & Merikangas, K. R. (2011). Social phobia and subtypes in the National Comorbidity Survey– Adolescent Supplement: Prevalence, correlates, and comorbidity. *Journal of the American Academy of Child &Adolescent Psychiatry, 50,* 870-880.

Calsyn, R. J., Winter, J. P., & Burger, G. K. (2005). The relationship between social anxiety and social support in adolescents. *A test of competing causal models. Adolescence, 40,* 103–113.

Davey, G. C. L. (2006). *Cognitive mechanisms in fear acquisition and maintenance.* Washington, DC: American Psychological Association.

Edelmann, R. J., Baker, S. R. (2002). Self-reported and actual physiological responses in social phobia. *British Journal of Clinical Psychology, 41,* 1-14.

Epkins, C. C. (2002). A Comparison of Two Self-Report Measures of Children's Social Anxiety in Clinic and Community Samples. *Journal of Clinical and Child and Adolescent Psychology, 31,* 69-79.

Essau, C. A., Conradt, J., & Petermann, F. (2009). Frequency and comorbidity and social fears in adolescents. *Behavior Research and Therapy*, 37, 831-843.

Fehm, L, & Pelissolo, A., (2005). Size and burden of social phobia in Europe. *European Neuropsychopharmacology* 15, 4, 453-462.

Gallagher, H. M., Rabian, B. A., McCloskey, M. S. (2004). A brief group cognitive behavioral intervention for social phobia in childhood. *Journal of Anxiety Disorders*, 18, 459-479.

Ginsburg, G. S., & Schlossberg, M. C. (2002). Family based treatment of childhood anxiety disorders. *International Review of Psychiatry*, 14, 143-154.

Groholt, B., Ekeberg, O., Wichstrom, L., & Haldorsen, T. (2000). Young suicide attempters: a comparison between a clinical and epidemiological sample. *Journal of the American Academy of Child and Adolescent Psychiatry*, 39, 868–875.

Gunnell, D., Hawton, K., Ho, D., Evans, J., O'Connor, S., Potokar, J., et al. (2008). Hospital admissions for self harm after discharge from psychiatric inpatient care: Cohort study. *British Medical Journal*, 337, 2278-91.

Hofmann, S. G., Asnaani, A., & Hinton, D. E. (2010). Cultural Aspects in Social Anxiety and Social Anxiety Disorder. *Depression and Anxiety*, 27, 1117–1127.

Hofmann, S. G.,& Asnaani, A., (2010). Cultural Aspects in Social Anxiety and Social Anxiety Disorder. *Depression and Anxiety*, 27, 1117–1127.

Kendler KS, Myers J, Prescott CA, Neale, M.C. (2001). The genetic epidemiology of irrational fears and phobias in men. Arch Gen Psychiatry 58:257-265.

Ollendick, H., & Hirshfeld-Becker, R.(2002). The developmental and psychopathology of social anxiety disorder. *Biological Psychiatry* 51. 1, 44-58.

Ranta, K., & Marttunen, M. (2009). Social phobia in Finnish general adolescent population: prevalence, Comorbidity, individual and family correlates, and service use. *Depression and Anxiety*, 26:528–536.

Tillfors, M., Furmark, T., Ekselius, L., & Fredrickson, M. (2001). Social phobia and avoidant personality disorder as related to parental history of social anxiety: a general population study. *Behaviour Research and Therapy*, 39, 289-298.

Turner, S. M., Beidel, D. C., & Borden, J. W., (2001). Social phobia: Axix I and II correlates. *Journal of Abnormal Psychology*, 100, 102-106.

YOUR KNOWLEDGE HAS VALUE

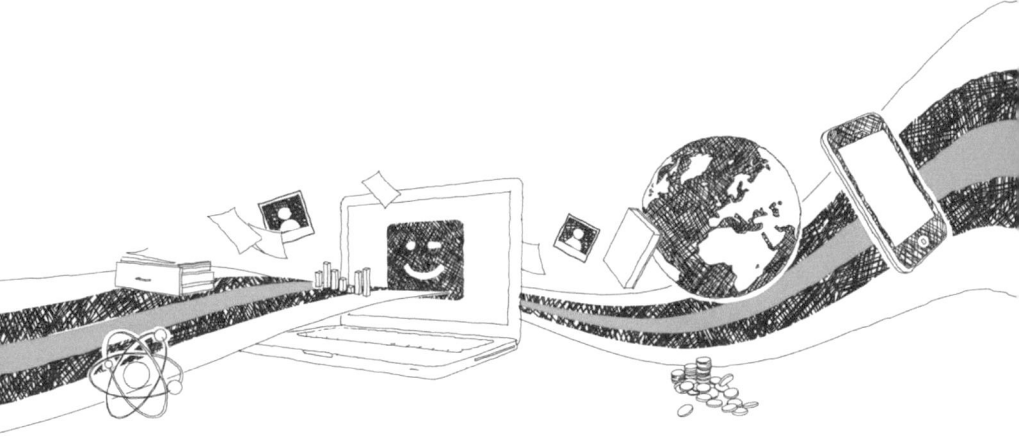

- We will publish your bachelor's and master's thesis, essays and papers

- Your own eBook and book - sold worldwide in all relevant shops

- Earn money with each sale

Upload your text at www.GRIN.com
and publish for free